Secrets
to a
Healthy Lifestyle

I0417296

7 Lifestyle Changes To Make
This Year the Best Yet

RON KNESS

Contents

Disclaimer

This publication is for informational purposes only and is not intended as medical advice. Medical advice should always be obtained from a qualified medical professional for any health conditions or symptoms associated with them.

Every possible effort has been made in preparing and researching this material. We make no warranties with respect to the accuracy, applicability of its contents or any omissions.

See your healthcare professional before starting any diet, health or exercise program!

Introduction

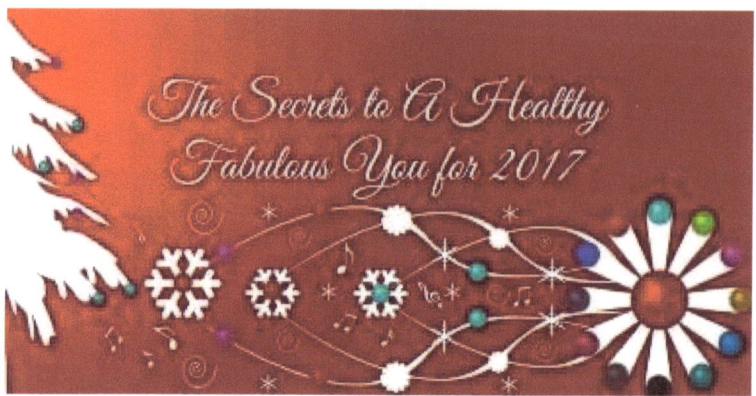

Along with a New Year comes the opportunity to let go of the past and start fresh and anew. It's a perfect time to get serious about getting healthy. Don't think of it as a new year's resolution. Think of it as a brand-new start on your life.

Out with the old, and in with the new. What's more is that it's not as difficult as you think. You can have less stress with a few simple daily actions, eat better by adding in more healthy food and get healthier by exercising more without feeling like it's so much work.

In addition, just a few money and time management changes will make all the difference in your life. Finally, you'll have more time for more fun without spending tons of money.

You're going to feel so much better with just a few specific changes, that you'll have the very best year you've ever had. Let's get started ….

Lower the Stress In Your Life

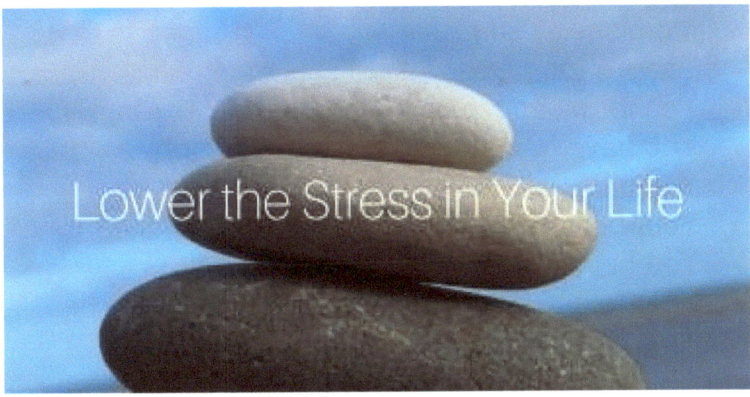

There are many factors that cause stress, both internal and external. Thankfully, for the most part, there are ways to limit exposure to stress and decrease the effects stress has on you that you can't control. There is no way to totally limit stress from your life. Some stress is good, too. You have good stress and bad stress. You have some stressors that you have control over and some that you do not.

Identify Stressors

Your first step to lowering your stress level is to first identify stressors you have in your life. Get out a piece of paper or a document on your computer and make a list of everything in your life that causes you stress. Don't worry yet if they're fixable, internal or external. Just write them all down.

Examples to get you started:

- You're always running late.
- You hate being stuck in traffic all the time.
- You're too tired to cook dinner at night.
- You're always losing things.
- You have family and friends who are difficult.
- You get frustrated getting dressed in the morning.

- You can't fix your hair the way you want to.
- Your kids are often late to school.
- Mornings are a nightmare.
- There's too much clutter in your home.
- You forget appointments.
- You have trouble paying bills each month.
- You hate your job.
- Your boss requires too much of you for the pay.
- You have too much work.
- Your health is not as good as you want it to be.

You get the idea. Write down anything that comes to mind. If you want to, take a week and write down anything that happens to you that causes stress every single day in that 7-day period.

Organize Your List

Once you have a good list, it's time to separate into internal and external. Pretty much everything that is internal should have a solution that's totally in your control. The things that are external you may only be able to control your own actions. But, there is still a lot you can do to lower the stress in your life.

Example:

Stressor	Internal	External
Running late	X	
Traffic		X
Too tired to cook	X	
You lose things	X	
Difficult family or friends		X
Too much clutter	X	
Horrible boss		X

Create Solutions

Now we can look at each stressor and come up with an appropriate solution. For example, if you're always running late for work or getting the kids to school, this is an internal issue. It's not controlled by outside forces and you're in complete control of it. It might not seem like it sometimes, but you are – and therefore you are able to make a change to it. One idea could be getting everyone up 30 minutes earlier.

Work Together

Have a family meeting about how you're all going to work together to make mornings better. Each night, ensure that everyone has their clothing laid out for the next day, including you; ensure everyone gets to bed on time so they are well rested in the morning; set alarms.

Teenagers can get themselves up and fed. Take that off your plate. If you prefer to ensure everyone eats healthy for breakfast, prepare it the night before, or let everyone eat fruit for breakfast. Fruit is the original fast food. Two or three bananas for breakfast is super healthy and better than a bowl of sugary cereal.

Let Go

If you take them to school, tell them what time you will be leaving each morning. Anyone not in the car at that time gets left behind. It will only take once or twice for your child to be left behind and then will them be on time the next time. It might sound controversial to let a teenager miss school, but ensure that there are other consequences such as you won't write them a note, and they don't get to do things they want to do if they don't go to school. If you do have access to school buses, start using them for even more freedom from this type of stress.

If you have younger children, get them ready for school first, and put them in front of the TV or computer game while you get ready. Don't hesitate to ask for help from your spouse. You can't expect a spouse to know what to do if you don't tell them and let them do it.

Don't micromanage them; it is not in your job description!. If everyone is in the car or at the bus stop on time, that's really the important thing. Everything else doesn't need to be perfect. Most school age children can dress themselves and should do so the minute they're able. This type of routine in the mornings does a couple other things – it builds a sense of responsibility and accountability in your child. A life skill that will serve them well throughout life.

Let's look at an external factor that you have no control over.

Traffic. One way to deal with traffic is to try other routes to work. There may even be a longer route that is quieter and maybe take less time. Even if it takes a little longer, less traffic is preferable and less stressful. If there is no other way, then you need to find another way to control your reaction to the traffic.

Listen to good music that makes you happy. Listen to a book that you wanted to read but don't have time to. This is going to be very helpful, because it makes being in the car something to look forward to rather than something to dread, even if traffic is not great. If you're a nervous driver, take steps to lessen that problem.

For example, don't have your first cup of coffee until after you get to work, since caffeine can heighten stress levels. Take a defensive driving course so that you know what to do in aggressive traffic. Ensure that your vehicle is the right one to drive in the type of traffic you need to navigate each day. That high gas mileage 3-cylinder car might not be made for driving in Atlanta traffic efficiently.

Eat Right to Reduce Stress

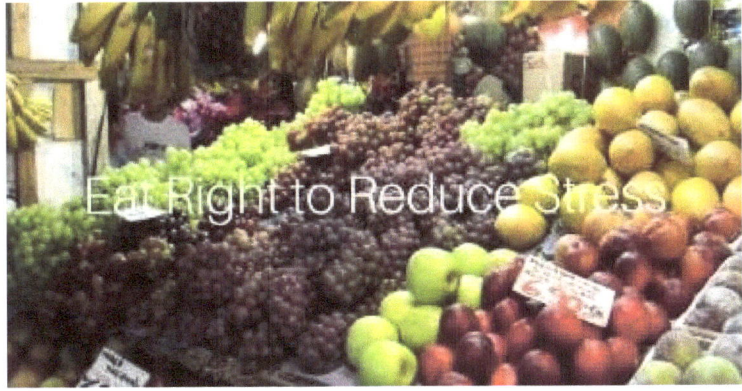

If you've heard it once, you've likely heard it 1000 times. Eating bad contributes to stress. It stresses your body so that you're not as healthy as you could be, and lack of health causes stomach issues, health issues, lack of energy and other problems. Here are 8 tips you can use to get more nutrition in your diet:

- **Limit Caffeine & Alcohol** – If you need caffeine to get through your day, you're addicted. The best thing to do is stop using it. Choose a time where you can take off work to go cold turkey or cut down slowly over a 30-day period. If you want to have a glass of wine at night after the kids go to bed, that's okay, but keep it to a normal 4-ounce serving size. Choose dryer wines to avoid a sugar kick. If you wake up with headaches or feeling dehydrated, you may want to limit your wine intake to one or two nights a week.

- **Create a Stress-Free Meal Environment** – Eating when everyone is rushed, yelling, and unhappy is not good for your digestion at all. Your home is supposed to be a safe place for every member of your family. Work hard to create that by keeping the TV off, making things easier by getting the whole family involved and talking with each other.

- Give children their own colored plates and cups that they can easily get out of the dishwasher to bring to the table to eat. Keep flatware in cups right on the table. Let kids load their own dish, plus one other. If everyone works together it makes life a lot easier.

- **Plan Your Meals Ahead of Time** – Meal planning is essential to success if you are committed to eating right. However you plan to eat, planning in advance will help. You can plan menus and use that as your shopping list yourself, or you can purchase a meal plan based on your needs. A couple of good meal planning sites are emeals.com, plantoeat.com, and wellvegan.com.

- **Don't Medicate with Food** – Some people use food like other people use drugs. If you find that you're stress eating at certain times of day instead of trying to fight the urge to eat, just replace your normal snack food with something healthy like fruit. There are rumors that fruit is bad for you, but most people, even diabetics, can find fruit to eat. Choose low sugar fruit like berries if you're worried about your blood sugar.

- **Stay Hydrated** – Drinking plenty of water and eating water-rich foods will ensure that you stay hydrated. How much you need to consume depends on factors such as climate, weight, body mass and more. But in general, the common suggestion of eight 8-ounce glasses of water a day is a good average to go by. But, if you're thirsty, you should drink.

- **Eat Whole Foods, Mostly Plants** – A low-fat, plant-based diet is recommended for maximum health. Eating this diet will naturally lead you to become the healthiest version of you. You'll lose weight, or gain weight if needed, lower your cholesterol and other signs of illness simply by following this way of eating.

Don't worry, it's simple to get enough of every nutrient you need eating a plant based diet.

- **Eat Enough Calories** – Everyone has a different caloric need which depends on your height, weight, muscle density, and activity level. In addition, health issues may affect your caloric needs. But, in general, women should eat at least 1500 calories a day and men about 2000 calories each day. Eating fewer can cause problems with having enough energy, headaches, and other signs and symptoms of a poor diet.

- **Take the Right Supplements** – Regardless of diet, today because we wash our food so well, and it doesn't contain as many nutrients as it did years ago, most people need to supplement their diet with vitamin B12. It can take a lot of years for a deficiency to show up, but it can cause permanent neurological damage, so it's super important. Ask your doctor if you should supplement and get yearly blood tests to be sure what you're doing is working for you.

Eating right is simple to do and totally in your control. If you have issues with getting meals on the table at night without pulling your hair out, you need a plan to follow. Create a menu that enables you to shop fewer times each month.

For example, go shopping every two weeks instead of weekly. Try to prepare some portions of your meals in advance so that at meal times you only mix a few ingredients together to make a meal. Example: Make a big pot of rice each week that can be combined with different ingredients to make meals such as rice and beans, stir-fry, wraps and other dishes.

If you can afford it, consider joining one of the meal delivery plans where the food comes to your door and you prepare it per the directions. Many of the meal delivery plans are very healthy, easy to prepare and can (for the right family) save money.

Get More Exercise

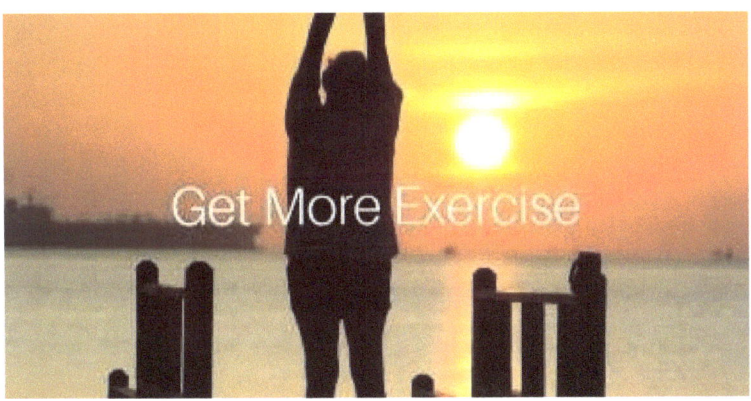

The word exercise often brings its own level of stress to people. Most people hate the word exercise and feel as if they have no time to do it anyway, much less the energy. But, intentional exercise is essential to good health. Good health helps lower stress levels. Therefore, instead of getting all worked up about working out, find ways to incorporate exercise into your daily routine.

- **Desk Exercises** – If you're stuck in a cubicle all day it can be hard to figure out how to get moving more. But, you can do exercises right at your desk. Tap your toes, squeeze your bottom, do Kegels, and move your arms – all while at the desk.

- **Take the Stairs** -- When you need to deliver a document to someone, take the long way, walk up the stairs – get in as many steps as you can rather than scanning and emailing. Not only will this help you physically, but getting more face time at work with people is always a good thing.

- **Walk at Lunch** – Grab a lunch that you can hold in your hands such as a smoothie or a wrap, and go for a walk.

Sit outside on a bench, enjoy your time outdoors even if it's cold outside. Just bundle up properly. The sunshine, even when it's cold, is good for you, as is the movement getting to the park bench and back (more steps).

- **Ask for a Standing Desk** – Some companies are starting to be aware of the dangers of sitting more than four hours a day. If you can get your company to spring for a sit/stand desk or at least standing stations, you'll save your health and everyone else's, too. Some people find that they're even more productive at a standing desk, as well.

- **TV Exercise** – Have a favorite show you like to watch? March in place while watching the show. In fact, anytime you want to watch a show, add some form of exercise to it, especially if you're a regular TV watcher. You can march in place, jog, do jumping jacks, pushups, sit-ups and other exercises and not miss a thing. Plus, you get built-in rest times in the form of commercials.

- **After Dinner Walk** – The after-dinner walk is a great way to not only get some extra steps in during the day, but is also a good way to connect with your children and/or your spouse. Plus, you can meet other walkers in your neighborhood, which is always a good thing to do. As studies show, more connection with neighbors, family and friends lowers stress.

- **Buy Experiences** – Instead of going out to eat or doing things that require little movement for fun, find things to do that cause you to move. Miniature golf, horseback riding, bike riding, roller skating and so forth area all fun experiences that you can pay for instead of paying for eating out.

You'll get more exercise, feel better, and be closer to each other, too. It's a win-win for sure.

- **Park at a Distance** – When going shopping or to work, park far from the door. You'll get in a few extra steps and have more energy just from that short walk to the door. Walking back to your car after shopping or working will also give you time to decompress from stress as you breathe in the fresh air on the way to your vehicle.

- **Waiting Movements** – You'll find that when you pay attention to your day, you're doing a lot of waiting. You wait for the microwave to beep, you wait for the printer at work, you wait for your kids to get to the car after school. Each of these moments is an opportunity to add more movement to your day. Squat in place, park away from the school and have kids walk to you while you walk the area as you wait.

Finally, remember to have fun. When you want to be with your family, try having experiences together that are active. After all, a day boogie boarding at the ocean or paddle boarding at the lake is more memorable and fun than sitting in front of screens all day. Sure, there is a place and time for sitting around and cuddling, but the more you move, the more you'll want to cuddle.

Incorporate Better Money Management

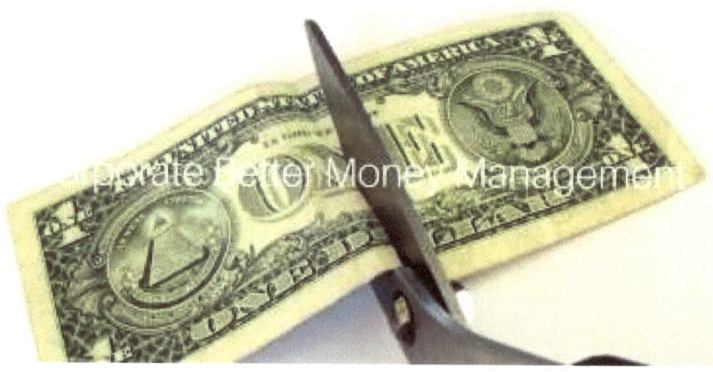

Many people identify money as a major cause of stress in their lives. Sometimes there are genuine reasons to feel stressed out about money. Being undereducated, underemployed, and underpaid can cause all sorts of stress. Not having enough money can make all other stressors seem even worse. Whether we like it or not, everyone needs money.

Money is important for shelter, food, and medical care. It not only helps you get healthy but stay healthy, because when you have enough money, you can pursue the things that are important, such as time with your family, eating healthy, and so forth. But, what's shocking is that people worry about money no matter how much they have. This suggests that the stress surrounding money isn't always really about dollars in and dollars out.

- **You Don't Need as Much as You Think** – Most people overspend because they think they need so many things.

But, if you really started only buying things because you truly need them, because they're useful, because they add value to your life, instead of you just think you need them or you want to impress someone else, you'd realize that you can do with a lot less. I mean really who needs dust-collecting knickknacks? No one.

- **Money Doesn't Make You Happy** – Okay let's get real. For most people, money can make you giggle a little – at most. But, true happiness comes from things that are free. The love of your spouse, the love of a parent, the love of friendship – these things can be had totally free. You only need to give of yourself. Beyond your basic financial needs, everything else is truly extra. Plus, study after study shows that owning less makes people happier.

- **Money Isn't The Best Contribution You Can Make** – Some people lament the money they don't have to give to special causes. But, you have something far more valuable that you can give to society and that's your time and attention. This is true with family and friends, too. Nothing is as important as giving of yourself to feel truly good about yourself.

- **Money Is Corrupting** – Often people don't realize how much of a pain it can be to have an enormous amount of money. It can corrupt the best people. People are happiest when they have enough to provide the basic comforts of life plus enough to save for the future and perhaps one good vacation a year. After that, most people get more stressed out.

Finally, when you can accept that money is a tool to help you live a happy, worry free life, you can then manage what you have and find ways to make more if you need it or buy less if you don't have it.

The biggest way you can affect the stress around money is to set a budget, stick to the budget, and plan for problems. Spend money on experiences and not things unless the things are truly things you need and will truly love.

Use Better Time Management

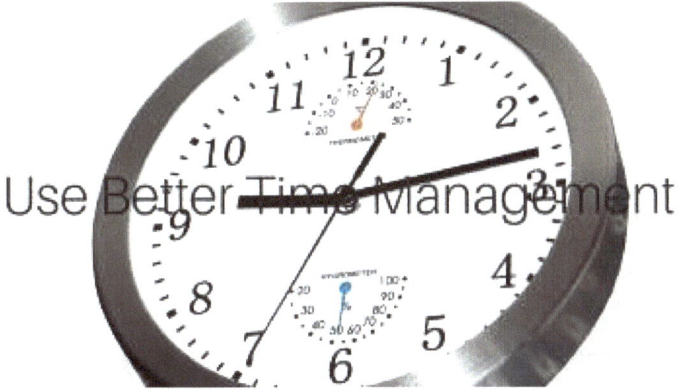

As mentioned early in this report, one stressor that people experience is feeling as if they don't have enough time. Time is one of those things that is equal for all people. Everyone has the same amount of time in each day. You cannot control time. All you can do is manage the time that you have better.

- **Schedule Everything** – Use a good calendar like Google Calendar to schedule every aspect of your day. Even if you plan to spend 2 hours reading a book, or 30 minutes walking with your daughter, write it down. By filling your calendar in this way, you'll be more likely to do what you say you will. Plus, it'll make it easier to say no about something when you look at how full your life already is.

- **Be Realistic About Time** – When you put entries into your calendar, ensure that you're giving enough time to get certain things done. If you need to go the store after work to get milk, how long will it really take? Don't say 10 minutes when you know in heavy traffic it's more like an hour.

- **Set a Time Limit** – For many projects and tasks, it's important to set a time limit so you don't keep doing it longer. Cleaning house, watching TV, sleeping, and exercising are all things that you can control the amount of time that you do them.

- **Give Yourself a Buffer** – Don't schedule things back to back. You're sure to get more stressed out and burned out. Instead build in a buffer in between different tasks. Try ten minutes, then if you find yourself bumping into time issues, increase it five minutes each time until you aren't having as many issues.

- **First Things First** – When you have a list of things to do, put it in order that makes sense. For example, if you need to run errands and grocery shop, don't shop first because that has to be last or at least before you go through the drive through to bring dinner home to your family.

- **Sleep 7 to 8 Hours Each Night** – This may seem like a strange thing to add when discussing time management but sleep is very important. Getting enough sleep, the right amount of sleep for you will help you work more efficiently each day.

- **Learn How to Say No** – Many people suffer great stress because they don't know how to say no to anyone. Being the go-to person for your friends, family and co-workers is admirable. However, it's also very difficult to maintain that level of involvement without ending up stressed out. You may not even be able to perform up to your own standards if you're overbooked.

- **Give Up Multitasking** – One of the most horrible habits people have today is multitasking. People even multitask when they drive now. The fact is that people do not perform well trying to do that. In truth, no one is capable of true multitasking. Your brain can only focus well on one thing at a time. Focus on each task that you need to do 100 percent and you'll find you do it better and faster.

- **Don't Try to Be Perfect** – Striving for perfection causes a lot of stress to many people all over the world. The sad fact is that perfection is impossible. The trick is learning when you've done your best and to stop and end a project instead of wasting time that won't produce additional results at least equal to the additional time invested.

- **Create New Habits** – Some things that help with time management are habits. For example, creating a weekly meal plan and grocery list can become a habit if you make it one. Going to bed each night at the same time so that you have more energy each day can also become a habit, as can other common activities that you must do. Be sure to allow at least 21 days to get a habit in place.

- **Avoid Too Much Screen Time** – Nothing can suck up time as much as computer and TV screens. They get in the way of intimacy with your family and friends. They interrupt and overcome your desire to exercise and get healthy. And, screens can get in the way of managing your time well so that you can lower your stress.

Time can seem like your worst enemy. But, if you learn to schedule everything in, including fun times, you'll soon be able to take advantage of time in productive ways. You may even find time to smell the roses.

Have More Fun

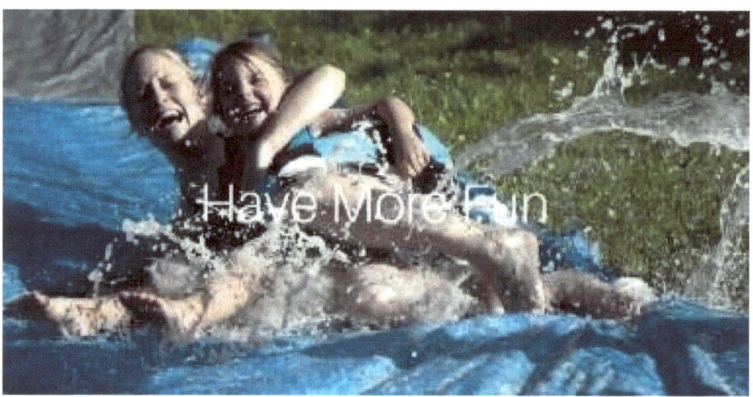

Life is supposed to be a fun adventure. It's not supposed to be all work and no play. When was the last time you truly had fun? When was the last time you laughed until you almost wet your pants? These are experiences that everyone should have, not only children. Having fun anchors the rest of your life and makes everything worth it.

- **Stop Worrying About What Others Think** – One huge impediment to fun is worrying about what other people think all the time. It's not that you need to do things that are controversial to have fun, it's just that for some people it's hard to be themselves. If you find yourself feeling that way, consider changing your thoughts and let yourself have fun.

- **You Don't Want to Spend Money** – Some people think the only way to have fun is to spend money. But that's not true. You can have plenty of fun without spending a dime. Play cards, go for a walk, play Frisbee, read a book together. Imagine what people did for fun before we had mass transportation, TV, and movies.

- **You're Not Sure How to Make Plans** – While it's good to make plans, not everything in the fun department has to be planned. You can have fun at the drop of a hat anyplace at any time if you can get yourself into the right frame of mind. Think positively, tell a joke, give someone a hug. Life is fun.

- **It's OK to Not Be Serious** – If you tend toward a serious personality, realize that you don't have to be serious all the time. It doesn't matter whether you're at home or at work. There are always opportunities to let your fun side shine through in appropriate ways.

- **Don't Wait for Perfection** – Sometimes planning to have fun can bring disappointment if you think it's going to be perfect. That family vacation to Disney will be a great memory for your kids, but will it be a good memory for you? Are you able to let go of the fact that tired kids will cry, whine and complain, even at Disney?

- **It Doesn't Have to Be Spectacular** – Another deterrent to having fun is thinking things need to be over the top to be fun. But, real fun doesn't have to be crazy, it should be natural and feel good. When you try to make things bigger and bigger you'll take away some of the fun.

- **Bring Back Date Night** – If you're married, have a significant other, or in another type of long-term relationship, it's imperative that you find time to spend together at least weekly without interruptions. Date night can be as simple as a picnic on your floor or you can go all out dress up and go out to dinner and movie or dinner and dancing. Even Karaoke if you dare.

- **Bring Back Family Game Night** – You can have a great time playing games with your family. Get out the board games, get out the old-fashioned cards and play games at least one night a week with your kids. Remember to be kind to teenagers and don't make game night Friday or Saturday night. Make it a weeknight. It only needs to be a couple of hours after dinner. Set a timer for games like Monopoly that can last longer and compute the winner based on accumulation by the time.

Kick Unhealthy Lifestyle Habits to the Curb

Limit or stop activities that can cause unhealthy lifestyle. In its place, do more productive and more important activities that will not affect your mood or be harmful to your health.

Stop or Limit Alcohol Intake – Even though red wine is proven to be good for the heart due to its resveratrol content, you still need to limit alcohol intake since too much of it can result into health and organ damages, e.g., heart weakening, liver problems, loss of sleep and feeling of tiredness. You can opt to totally stop drinking and get resveratrol pills instead.

Stop drug use and abuse – Aside from those prescribed, it comes as no secret that dangerous drugs can lead to many unhealthy results some of which are fatal. It can give your body an incredible amount of toxin that can immediately weaken the immune system of your body that you need to fight illnesses.

Have safe sex – one good exercise that can bring positive results is having sex. To make sure you do not get sick from it, do it with your wife, husband or only one partner. Sex can bring you more energy, reduce your cholesterol in the body, increase oxygen flow to the brains, help you get more sleep, reduce stress and pressures and even serve as a natural pain reliever, if you do it smart.

Give up smoking – You can reduce health issues, like heart and lung disease, by quitting altogether and have more money to do other healthier things.

Final Thoughts

Finally, just find ways to laugh more. Laughing is not only wonderful exercise, it boosts endorphins and makes you happy. The more you can laugh, the more fun you will have doing even "boring" things. For example, even grocery shopping alone with your spouse can be fun if you make a day of it.

Did you know that world renowned medical centers teach that laughing makes you live longer? That's because laughter relaxes you. It lets the body rid itself of that internal turmoil caused by the stress of your days.

Even if you're a pessimistic person, you can still benefit from humor. Whether that humor is found in laughing at silly jokes or in watching television that tickles your funny bone, the chortles can help your body fight the aging process.

Endorphins are one of your body's defensive weapons against diseases. By raising up a standard and relieving stress, this chemical strives to keep your blood pressure at its heart healthy best and also fights a battle against physical problems that can lead to heart attacks.

You might not have known that laughter can also give you a stronger immune system. You'll also have more energy and discover that regular bouts of merriment helps to lessen pain whether physical or emotional.

Laughing makes you live longer and lets you look good while you're living! Laughter causes feeling of happiness, gives you a sense of wellbeing. When you're happy, it shows up on your skin.

Because you're more relaxed, you'll look and feel ten times younger. But you can put the stress to the test. Look at photos of people in extremely stressful, high profile jobs. Take a glance at their photos before they started the job and then one year to two years later and you can see how the stress has aged them.

But even if you're not in a particularly high stress job or you don't have a high stress life, you can still get the rewards that laughing can give you. Laughter can give you the mental fortitude to handle people that aren't easy to be around.

It can also help you be more prepared to roll with life's punches. Look for the humor in every stressful situation you encounter and you'll be adding years to your life. While it's true that laughing makes you live longer, that doesn't mean that you should ignore all the good health rules that you know bring you benefit.

Rules like eating healthy, getting plenty of rest and staying in the best physical shape that you possibly can are rules you shouldn't ignore. Join in the fight to feel and look your best by taking your vitamins and supplements and keep your skin looking good by investing in quality anti-aging creams and lotions.

Turn off electronics, head for a walk in the park, have a picnic, then go grocery shopping leisurely. Make fun a priority in your life and you'll naturally be healthier, happier and have an amazing year, every year.

Other Relevant Books by This Author

If you would like to read more relevant books about this topic, here is a list of the CreateSpace links, titles and descriptions from this author:

https://www.createspace.com/6410557

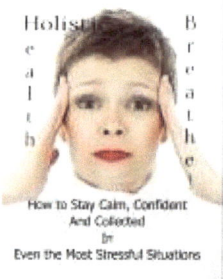

Ron Kness

Breathe!: How to Stay Calm, Confident and Collected In Even the Most Stressful Situations

The objective is not to completely eliminate stress or anxiety. This is something we need to make clear right from the very start.

Believe it or not, stress and anxiety are actually useful emotions. Both put the body into a physiological state of heightened arousal, attention and awareness and can even increase physical strength and power. When you're stressed, you're essentially 'amped up' and this makes you better at completing physical tasks or reacting on the spot.

Psychologists have also shown that stress can be a positive motivating force in the right circumstances. Stress is what compels us to study for exams and what motivates us to save money as a contingency fund. Specifically, this type of stress is known as 'eustress' and is a very useful phenomenon.

The problem is that many of us have no control over when we become stressed or when we get anxiety. This then in turn leads to us feeling those emotions in maladaptive situations.

Being chased by a lion? Then yes, the fight or flight response as it is known is exactly what you need.
About to give a big speech to a large audience? Then the same response is going to make you look nervous and unconfident.

Likewise, it's important that the stress response be appropriate to the situation that we're in. Being a little stressed in a crowd is normal – but having such a powerful response that you end up having a panic attack and fainting is a problem.

So our objective here is not to remove stress entirely but simply to learn to control it, to hone it and to use it to our advantage.

That's what this book is all about. This book will teach you to take control of your physiology and your psychology so that you can experience the right emotion when you need it. You can suppress your fight-or-flight response during a presentation in order to come across as calm and collected and you can switch it on again during competition so that you become an unstoppable athlete.

You might not think that you currently have a particular problem with stress and this may well be true. But even if you don't experience any crippling anxiety, that doesn't mean you couldn't benefit from being more calm, more collected and more in control of your thoughts and feelings. All of us experience inappropriate anxiety to some extent, the question is simply where you fall on that spectrum.

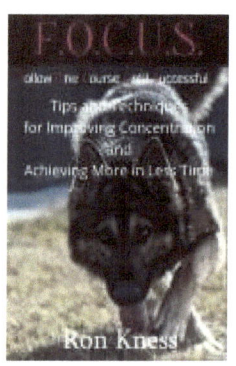

F.O.C.U.S. - Follow One Course Until Successful: Tips and Techniques for Improving Your Concentration and Achieving More in Less Time

Do you seem to get less done, but are more "busy" than the year before? Every year our attention span goes down; in 2015 it dropped to a low of 8.5 seconds compared to 12 seconds in 2000.

As each year goes by we're having more and more difficulty focusing on one thing at a time. And when we finally can start to focus, something always ends up pulling us away. I get it - everyone's always busy, but never seems to be able to get enough done!

In my book F.O.C.U.S. - Follow One Course Until Successful, I talk about tips and techniques you can implement today that will help you focus on one thing at a time which enables you to get more done in a day than you are presently doing

.

https://www.createspace.com/6794823

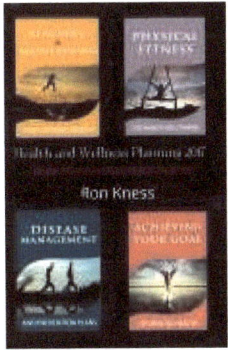

Health and Wellness Planning - 2017: 4 Reports to Help Make This Your Healthiest Year Yet

Your doctor is a valuable resource when it comes to your health and fitness concerns. However, many people don't know how to talk to their doctors.

After some visits, you might even leave the doctor's office with more questions than answers. Maybe you feel that you don't have a chance during your appointment to say what's really on your mind.

Talking to your doctor is very important before you begin any new fitness and exercise regimen, especially if you have been quite sedentary up until now. Here are some tips to help you prepare so you can leave your next appointment with the best answers possible.

- Bring up the topic of fitness and exercise yourself. If you wait for your doctor to mention it, the subject may not come up. Some doctors are reluctant to bring up fitness and exercise because they don't want to hurt their patients' feelings.

- Prepare your questions ahead of time. Your doctor has budgeted only a certain amount of time to spend with you. You can make your appointment run more quickly and smoothly by writing down your questions ahead of time. When your appointment starts, let your doctor know that you have a list of questions. That will indicate to your doctor that you are seeking particular information and they will usually give you the opportunity to work your way through the list.

- Ask about what kinds of exercise you should be doing. Your doctor will know your medical history and will know if certain types of exercise would be unwise for you to try. They may be concerned about you getting injured. As well, if you have any medical conditions or are taking any medications, that might affect your ability to do certain exercises.

- Ask about your resting heart rate and what your target heart rate should be. Your doctor can explain these to you. Your doctor will be able to tell you what your target heart rate should be based on your age and medical condition. He or she can also show you how to easily calculate your heart rate.

- If you want to lose weight, this is a good opportunity to discuss a reasonable weight-loss goal with your doctor. He or she will be able to tell you what a realistic weight loss would be for your condition. They can also help you determine your ideal weight.

- Ask about diet and nutrition. Your doctor can tell you how many calories you should be eating each day to stay healthy and may recommend certain foods to improve and maintain your health.

- Take notes. While your doctor is speaking, take notes of their answers. With so much information being thrown at you, it will be impossible to remember all of it. You may also want to bring along a friend to ask any questions you didn't think of and to help remind you of important details after you leave.

Your doctor is an important partner in your health care. By taking this advice, you will be able to start a meaningful conversation with your doctor and gain helpful information.

In this book are four reports that after reading may help you better plan your next trip with your doctor in regard to health and fitness:
• Achieving Your Goal of Mental Health
• Disease Management and Prevention Plans
• Physical Fitness for Energy and Stamina
• Reaching and Maintaining Your Optimal Weight

These 4 reports will not only help you improve your health and wellness, but also serve to spur meaningful conversations with your doctor.

About the Author

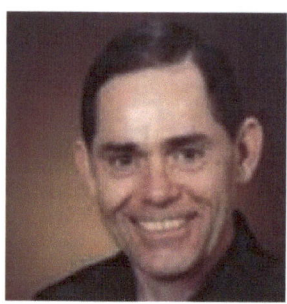

I grew up in Central Minnesota, where my parents owned and operated a fishing resort. Once out of high school I tried a couple of semesters of college, only to quit halfway through the Spring term; I decided at that time that college wasn't for me.

Then I decided to follow my father's previous occupation as an auto mechanic. I graduated from a two-year of vocational training course and worked as a mechanic for five years. While in vocational training, I decided to join the National Guard where I eventually ended up working full-time for 32 years.

So how does all of this relate to writing? In one of my leadership schools, the instructor, who was an English teacher at a juvenile detention center, presented writing to me in a whole new way - a way that started to develop my interest in working with words.

I eventually went back to college on the GI Bill while I was working and earned my Bachelor's degree in Business Administration. Taking a class or two per semester at night and on weekends took me seven years to complete my degree.

Fast forward about 40 years and I now have published over 75 books on Amazon for Kindle, CreateSpace and other publishing platforms.

Besides my own writing, I also ghostwrite ebooks, reports, articles, blogs and do Kindle conversions for clients on a variety of topics.

Today my wife and I are retired from our careers and live in Gold Canyon, AZ. I now write as a retirement business where you'll find me happily sitting in my office typing away on my laptop as I work on my next book or ghostwriting project . . . that is if we are not traveling on a cruise ship - our new-found mode of travel.

www.ingramcontent.com/pod-product-compliance
Lightning Source LLC
Chambersburg PA
CBHW050903290526

45792CB00002B/689